The Ult

Galveston Diet Cookbook for

Beginners 2023

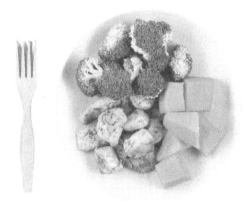

*60 Wholesome, Budget-friendly and Easy Vegetarian
Recipes to Burn Fat and Tame Hormonal Symptoms.*

By

Dr. Lucy Mogen

Copyright © 2023 by Lucy Mogen

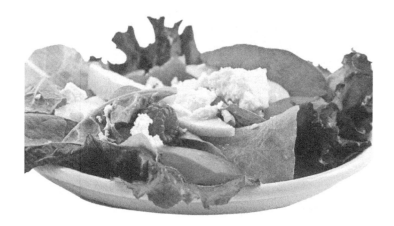

Table of Contents

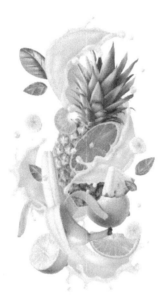

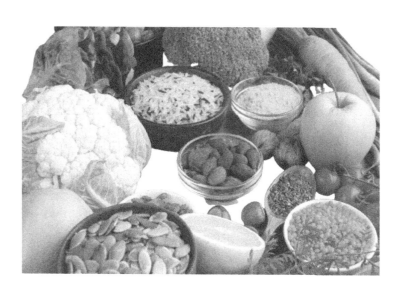

Introduction to the Vegetarian Galveston Diet

Welcome to the world of the Vegetarian Galveston Diet, where health meets deliciousness and vitality. In today's fast-paced world, finding a sustainable and nourishing dietary approach is key, and the Vegetarian Galveston Diet is here to guide you towards optimal well-being.

Did you know that obesity rates have been steadily rising in the United States, with over 42% of adults classified as obese? Alongside this, hormonal imbalances are increasingly prevalent, affecting women's health in various ways. It's clear that a holistic approach to health is essential, and that's where the Vegetarian Galveston Diet shines.

Imagine Amber, a vibrant woman in her 30s who struggled with excess weight and hormonal fluctuations for years. Frustrated by the lack of sustainable solutions, she discovered the Vegetarian Galveston Diet. Through adopting this approach, Amber not only shed unwanted pounds but also regained hormonal balance, leading to increased energy and an overall sense of well-being. Her story resonates with countless individuals seeking a natural path to health.

The Vegetarian Galveston Diet combines the powerful principles of the Galveston Diet with the benefits of a plant-based lifestyle. This diet focuses on whole, nutrient-dense foods while avoiding processed ingredients and harmful additives. By embracing a vegetarian approach, you'll not only support your body's hormonal balance but also nourish it with plant-based proteins, fiber, vitamins, and minerals.

Whether you're looking to shed excess weight, regain hormonal equilibrium, or simply boost your overall health, the Vegetarian Galveston Diet is your guide. With this cookbook, you'll discover a diverse range of recipes that tantalize your taste buds while supporting your well-being. From nourishing breakfasts to vibrant lunches, satisfying dinners, and delectable desserts, each dish is thoughtfully crafted to align with the Galveston Diet principles and the benefits of a vegetarian lifestyle.

Get ready to embark on a journey that redefines your relationship with food and health. The Vegetarian Galveston Diet isn't just a diet; it's a lifestyle that empowers you to take charge of your well-being and embrace vitality. Join us as we explore the wonderful world of nutrient-packed, flavor-rich meals that nourish both body and soul. **Your health journey begins here!**

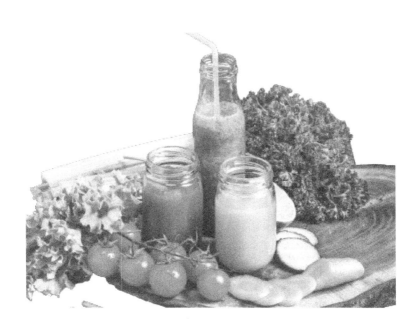

Chapter One

Understanding the Galveston Diet Principles

The Galveston Diet, renowned for its holistic approach to health and weight management, has now embraced the realm of vegetarianism, extending its benefits to a wider audience. Delving into the heart of this dietary philosophy, we uncover the core principles that make the Vegetarian Galveston Diet an appealing and effective choice for those seeking wellness through plant-based nutrition.

Benefits of a Vegetarian Approach

Hormonal Balance and Weight Management: Within the Vegetarian Galveston Diet, the focus on plant-based whole foods aids in hormone regulation, stimulating weight loss, and overall well-being. Processed and inflammatory foods are avoided, enhancing your body's natural ability to balance hormones and manage weight effectively.

Cardiovascular Health and Disease Prevention: By adopting a vegetarian path within the Galveston Diet, you're reducing the consumption of saturated fats and cholesterol often associated with animal products. This supports heart health and decreases the risk of chronic diseases.

Gut Health and Digestion: A plant-based diet rich in fiber, fruits, vegetables, and whole grains nurtures a healthy gut microbiome. Improved digestion leads to enhanced nutrient absorption and overall well-being.

Sustainability: Choosing a vegetarian approach contributes to sustainable living by reducing carbon footprints and promoting a kinder impact on the environment.

Navigating Your Vegetarian Galveston Diet Journey

Selecting Nutrient-Dense Foods: Discover the wide array of plant-based options that align with the Galveston Diet's principles. Learn how nutrient-dense vegetables, legumes, whole grains, nuts, and seeds can nourish your body.

Creating Balanced Meals: Master the art of combining food groups for balanced plates that fuel your body. Find the ideal balance of carbohydrates, proteins, healthy fats, and fiber for sustained energy and optimal digestion.

Mindful Eating and Portion Control: Develop a mindful eating practice that connects you with your body's hunger and fullness cues. Understand portion control to support digestive efficiency and energy levels.

Incorporating Vegetarian Galveston Diet into Your Lifestyle

Adapting Favorite Recipes: Learn how to transform your favorite recipes to fit the vegetarian framework. Discover ingredient substitutions, cooking techniques, and creative ideas that celebrate plant-based abundance.

Balanced Nutrition and Wellness: The Vegetarian Galveston Diet isn't just about weight loss; it's about holistic well-being. Embrace the power of balanced nutrition to support vitality, mental clarity, and overall health.

Culinary Exploration: Venture into the world of plant-based culinary arts. Embrace diversity by exploring a variety of plant-based foods, flavors, and cuisines that align with the Galveston Diet's principles.

By embracing the Galveston Diet's vegetarian approach, you embark on a holistic voyage towards optimal well-being. It's not just about shedding pounds; it's about revitalizing your relationship with food, nurturing your body, and experiencing the transformative power of balanced nutrition. As you venture further into this section, you'll find yourself equipped with the knowledge and inspiration needed to embark on a fulfilling Vegetarian Galveston Diet journey that positively impacts every facet of your life.

Embarking on your Vegetarian Galveston Diet journey requires understanding the nuances of your new culinary approach. We provide you with a comprehensive guide to selecting the right foods to support your hormonal balance and weight management goals. From nutrient-dense vegetables to plant-based proteins, discover how to create satisfying meals that fuel your body while enhancing your well-being.

Learn how to artfully combine various food groups to create a balanced plate that aligns with the Galveston Diet's principles. Dive into the world of mindful eating and understand the importance of listening to your body's cues. We guide you through portion control, helping you strike the perfect balance to optimize digestion and sustain energy levels throughout the day.

Incorporating Vegetarian Galveston Diet into Your Lifestyle

The Vegetarian Galveston Diet isn't just a dietary plan – it's a lifestyle shift that empowers you to take charge of your health and enjoy nourishing foods that support your journey. Discover creative ways to adapt your favorite recipes to fit the vegetarian framework. We provide you with cooking tips, ingredient substitutions, and innovative culinary ideas that celebrate the abundance of plant-based options available.

By embracing the Galveston Diet's vegetarian approach, you embark on a holistic voyage towards optimal well-being. It's not just about shedding pounds; it's about revitalizing your relationship with food, nurturing your body, and experiencing the transformative power of balanced nutrition. As you venture further into this section, you'll find yourself equipped with the knowledge and inspiration needed to embark on a fulfilling Vegetarian Galveston Diet journey that positively impacts every facet of your life.

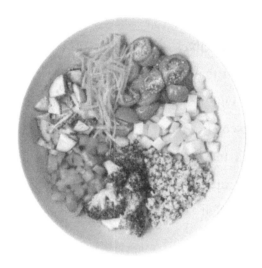

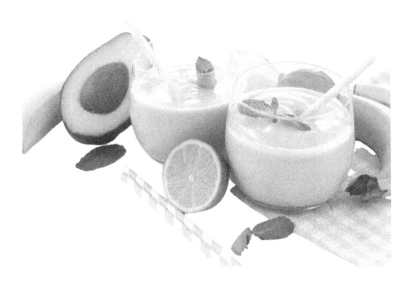

Chapter Two

Boosting Digestive Wellness: Nourishing Your Gut with Plant-Based Power

The symphony of life within us thrives when our digestive system is in harmony. From the absorption of nutrients to the strength of our immune defenses, the gut plays a pivotal role. For followers of the Vegetarian Galveston Diet, the path to vibrant health flows through the conscious selection of plant-based foods that nurture digestive well-being. This chapter delves deep into the realm of gut-healing foods, and the essential roles prebiotics, probiotics, and fiber-rich choices play in maintaining a thriving digestive ecosystem.

Gut-Healing Foods for Vegetarians

Every bite can be a step towards better digestion. Plant-based eating offers an array of ingredients that invigorate the gut and boost overall vitality.

Fermented Delights: Fermented foods are brimming with beneficial bacteria that bolster the gut. Sauerkraut, kimchi, kefir, and tempeh introduce friendly probiotics, enhancing digestion and aiding nutrient absorption.

Herbaceous Heroes: Nature's remedies abound in ginger, turmeric, and peppermint. These herbs possess anti-inflammatory properties that soothe the digestive tract, alleviate discomfort, and encourage smoother digestion.

Nutrient-Rich Produce: The bounty of plant-based foods like bananas, avocados, and leafy greens is a gift to the gut. Rich in fiber, vitamins, and antioxidants, they support a healthy gut lining and overall digestive well-being.

Prebiotics, Probiotics, and Fiber-Rich Choices

The dynamic trio of prebiotics, probiotics, and fiber acts as guardians of your gut. They ensure a thriving microbial community, robust immune responses, and efficient nutrient absorption.

Fiber for Gut Health: Whole grains, legumes, fruits, and vegetables are abundant in soluble and insoluble fiber. These fibers act as prebiotics, feeding the beneficial gut bacteria and promoting regularity.

Probiotic-Rich Foods: The world of plant-based probiotics includes yogurt, kefir, miso, and kombucha. These living foods introduce friendly bacteria, enhancing gut diversity and defense mechanisms.

Prebiotic-Containing Foods: Onions, garlic, leeks, chicory root, and Jerusalem artichokes contain prebiotics that serve as nourishment for gut microbes. They encourage the growth of beneficial bacteria and contribute to gut balance.

By weaving these plant-powered choices into your daily meals, you're nurturing a resilient digestive system. As you explore the interplay between gut-healing foods, prebiotics, probiotics, and fiber, you'll unlock the potential to enhance nutrient absorption and foster a balanced gut microbiome.

Remember, the journey to optimal digestive wellness is a gradual one. Savor each culinary adventure and listen to your body's cues. As you infuse your Vegetarian Galveston Diet with gut-loving selections, you're not just nourishing your body—you're kindling a radiant sense of vitality that radiates from within. It's a journey that embraces nourishment in every sense and promises lasting benefits for your overall well-being.

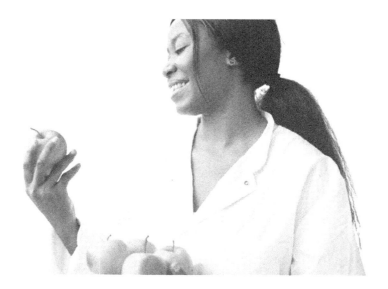

Chapter Three

Rise and Shine: Wholesome Vegetarian Galveston Breakfast Recipes

1. Creamy Chia Pudding

Ingredients:

- 3 tbsp chia seeds

- 1 cup almond milk (unsweetened)

- 1 tsp vanilla extract

- Fresh berries for topping

Instructions:

- In a bowl, mix chia seeds, almond milk, and vanilla extract.

- Stir well and refrigerate overnight.

- In the morning, give it a good stir, and top with fresh berries before serving.

2. *Veggie Omelette*

Ingredients:

- 2 eggs (or egg substitute)

- 1/4 cup diced bell peppers

- 1/4 cup diced tomatoes

- 1/4 cup chopped spinach

- Salt and pepper to taste

- Olive oil for cooking

Instructions:

- Add salt and pepper to a bowl of whisked eggs.

- Heat olive oil in a pan, add diced veggies, and sauté until tender.

- Pour whisked eggs over the veggies and cook until set.

- Cook the omelette for a further few minutes after folding it in half.

3. *Nutty Overnight Oats*

Ingredients:

- 1/2 cup rolled oats

- 1/2 cup almond milk (unsweetened)

- 1 tbsp chia seeds

- 1 tbsp chopped nuts (almonds, walnuts)

- 1 tsp honey or maple syrup (optional)

- Sliced bananas for topping

Instructions:

- In a jar, mix chia seeds, almond milk, and oats.

- Refrigerate overnight.

- In the morning, top with chopped nuts and sliced bananas. If desired, drizzle with honey or maple syrup.

4. Greek Yogurt Parfait

Ingredients:

- 1/2 cup Greek yogurt (unsweetened)

- 1/4 cup granola (low-sugar)

- 1/4 cup mixed berries

- 1 tbsp honey

Instructions:

- Greek yogurt, granola, and mixed berries should be layered in a glass.

- Drizzle with honey on top.

5. *Avocado Toast*

Ingredients:

- 1 whole-grain toast

- 1/2 avocado, mashed

- Salt and pepper to taste

- Red pepper flakes (optional)

- Sliced radishes for topping

Instructions:

- Toast the bread.

- On top of the toast, spread the mashed avocado.

- Add salt, pepper, and red pepper flakes for seasoning.

- Top with sliced radishes.

6. *Blueberry Banana Smoothie*

Ingredients:

- 1 banana
- 1/2 cup blueberries
- 1 cup spinach leaves
- 1/2 cup almond milk (unsweetened)
- 1/4 cup water

Instructions:

- Blend all ingredients until smooth.

7. Quinoa Breakfast Bowl

Ingredients:

- 1/2 cup cooked quinoa
- 1/4 cup mixed nuts and seeds
- 1/4 cup chopped fresh fruit (like mango or kiwi)
- 1/4 cup coconut flakes
- 1 tbsp nut butter

Instructions:

- In a bowl, layer cooked quinoa, nuts, seeds, chopped fruit, and coconut flakes.

- Drizzle with nut butter.

8. *Almond Butter Banana Toast*

Ingredients:

- 1 slice whole-grain bread

- 1 tbsp almond butter

- 1/2 banana, sliced

Instructions:

- Toast the bread.

- Spread almond butter on top.

- Arrange banana slices on the almond butter.

9. Spinach and Mushroom Scramble

Ingredients:

- 2 eggs (or egg substitute)

- 1/4 cup chopped spinach

- 1/4 cup sliced mushrooms

- Salt and pepper to taste

- Olive oil for cooking

Instructions:

- Heat olive oil in a pan, add sliced mushrooms and sauté until golden.

- Add chopped spinach and cook until wilted.

- Whisk eggs in a bowl, pour into the pan, and scramble with veggies.

- Season with salt and pepper.

10. Fruit Salad

Ingredients:

- Assorted fresh fruits (berries, melon, grapes, etc.)

- Instructions:

- Wash and chop fruits.

- Mix them together in a bowl to create a colorful and refreshing fruit salad.

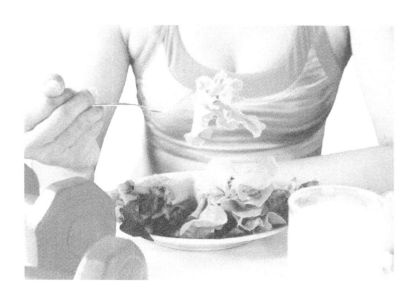

Chapter Four

Midday Delights: Nourishing Vegetarian Galveston Lunch and Light Meals

1. Mediterranean Chickpea Salad

Ingredients:

- 2 cups cooked chickpeas

- 1 cup cherry tomatoes, halved

- 1 cup cucumber, diced

- 1/2 cup red onion, thinly sliced

- 1/2 cup Kalamata olives, chopped

- 1/4 cup crumbled feta cheese

- 2 tablespoons extra-virgin olive oil

- Juice of 1 lemon

- Fresh parsley for garnish

Instructions:

- Chickpeas, cherry tomatoes, cucumber, red onion, Kalamata olives, and feta cheese crumbles should all be combined in a big bowl.
- Lemon juice and extra virgin olive oil should be drizzled on.
- Toss well to combine and garnish with fresh parsley before serving.

2. *Quinoa and Avocado Salad*

Ingredients:

- 2 cups cooked quinoa

- 1 ripe avocado, diced

- 1 cup baby spinach

- 1/2 cup diced red bell pepper

- 1/4 cup chopped red onion

- 2 tablespoons chopped fresh cilantro

- Juice of 1 lime

- Salt and pepper to taste

Instructions:

- In a bowl, combine cooked quinoa, diced avocado, baby spinach, diced red bell pepper, chopped red onion, and fresh cilantro.

- Add salt and pepper, then drizzle with lime juice.

- Toss gently to mix all ingredients, and serve.

3. Caprese Salad Wrap

Ingredients:

- 4 large whole wheat tortillas

- 2 cups baby spinach

- 1 cup cherry tomatoes, halved

- 1 cup fresh mozzarella, cubed

- Fresh basil leaves

- Balsamic glaze

Instructions:

- Lay out each tortilla and layer with baby spinach, cherry tomatoes, fresh mozzarella, and basil leaves.

- Drizzle with balsamic glaze.

- Roll up the tortillas into wraps and serve.

4. Roasted Vegetable and Hummus Wrap

Ingredients:

- 4 large whole wheat tortillas

- 2 cups of roasted mixed veggies, including bell peppers, eggplant, zucchini, etc.

- 1 cup hummus

- Fresh spinach leaves

Instructions:

- Lay out each tortilla and spread a layer of hummus.

- Add a handful of fresh spinach leaves and roasted vegetables.

- Roll up the tortillas into wraps and serve.

5. *Greek Salad with Tofu*

Ingredients:

- 1 block extra-firm tofu, cubed

- 4 cups mixed greens

- 1 cup diced cucumber

- 1/2 cup diced red onion

- 1/2 cup Kalamata olives, chopped

- 1/4 cup crumbled feta cheese

- Greek dressing (olive oil, lemon juice, oregano)

Instructions:

- Preheat oven to 375°F (190°C).

- Place tofu cubes on a baking sheet and bake until golden and slightly crispy.

- In a large bowl, combine mixed greens, diced cucumber, red onion, Kalamata olives, and crumbled feta cheese.

- Top with baked tofu and drizzle with Greek dressing.

6. Spinach and Chickpea Buddha Bowl

Ingredients:

- 2 cups cooked quinoa

- 1 cup cooked chickpeas

- 2 cups fresh spinach leaves

- 1/2 cup grated carrot

- 1/4 cup sliced red cabbage

- 1/4 cup sliced almonds

- Creamy tahini dressing

Instructions:

- In a bowl, layer cooked quinoa, cooked chickpeas, fresh spinach leaves, grated carrot, and sliced red cabbage.

- Drizzle with creamy tahini dressing and sprinkle with sliced almonds.

7. *Stuffed Bell Peppers*

Ingredients:

- 4 large bell peppers, cut in half, with seeds removed

- 2 cups cooked brown rice

- 1 cup black beans, drained and rinsed

- 1 cup corn kernels (fresh or frozen)

- 1 cup diced tomatoes

- 1/2 cup shredded vegan cheese

- 1 teaspoon chili powder

- 1/2 teaspoon cumin

- Salt and pepper to taste

Instructions:

- Preheat the oven to 375°F (190°C).

- In a bowl, mix cooked brown rice, black beans, corn, diced tomatoes, vegan cheese, chili powder, cumin, salt, and pepper.

- The mixture should be placed inside each bell pepper half.

- Place the stuffed bell peppers on a baking sheet and bake for about 20-25 minutes, until peppers are tender.

8. *Lentil and Vegetable Stir-Fry*

Ingredients:

- 2 cups cooked green lentils

- 2 cups mixed stir-fry vegetables (broccoli, bell peppers, snap peas, carrots, etc.)

- 1/4 cup low-sodium soy sauce

- 2 tablespoons sesame oil

- 1 tablespoon minced ginger

- 1 tablespoon minced garlic

- 1 teaspoon red pepper flakes (optional)

Instructions:

- Sesame oil should be heated over medium-high heat in a large skillet.

- Add minced ginger and garlic, and sauté for a minute.

- Add mixed stir-fry vegetables and cook until they start to soften.

- Add cooked green lentils, soy sauce, and red pepper flakes (if using).

- Stir-fry for a few minutes, or until the ingredients are thoroughly blended and cooked.

9. *Sweet Potato and Black Bean Salad*

Ingredients:

- 2 medium sweet potatoes, cubed and roasted

- 1 cup black beans, drained and rinsed

- 1 cup chopped kale or spinach

- 1/4 cup chopped red onion

- 1/4 cup chopped cilantro

- Juice of 1 lime

- 2 tablespoons olive oil

- Salt and pepper to taste

Instructions:

- In a bowl, combine roasted sweet potato cubes, black beans, chopped kale or spinach, red onion, and cilantro.

- Drizzle with lime juice and olive oil.

- Add salt and pepper, then gently toss to combine..

10. Curried Chickpea Salad Wraps

Ingredients:

- 2 cups cooked chickpeas

- 1/2 cup chopped celery

- 1/4 cup chopped red onion

- 1/4 cup chopped fresh cilantro

- 1/4 cup vegan mayo

- 2 teaspoons curry powder

- Salt and pepper to taste

- Large lettuce leaves for wrapping

Instructions:

- In a bowl, mash half of the cooked chickpeas with a fork.

- Add chopped celery, red onion, cilantro, vegan mayo, curry powder, salt, and pepper.

- Mix well and fold in the remaining whole chickpeas.

- Spoon the chickpea salad onto large lettuce leaves, wrap, and enjoy.

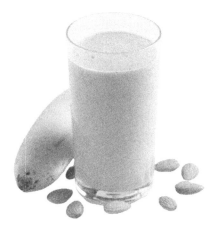

Chapter Five

Evening Feasts: Savory Vegetarian Galveston Dinner Recipes

1. Quinoa-Stuffed Bell Peppers

Ingredients:

- 4 large bell peppers

- 1 cup cooked quinoa

- 1 cup black beans, cooked and drained

- 1 cup corn kernels

- 1 cup diced tomatoes

- 1 cup shredded vegan cheese

- 1 teaspoon ground cumin

- 1 teaspoon paprika

- Salt and pepper to taste

Instructions:

- Preheat the oven to 375°F (190°C).

- Take the bell peppers' tops off and scoop out the seeds.

- In a bowl, combine cooked quinoa, black beans, corn kernels, diced tomatoes, shredded vegan cheese, ground cumin, paprika, salt, and pepper.

- Stuff the mixture into the bell peppers.

- Place the stuffed bell peppers in a baking dish and cover with aluminum foil.

- Bake the peppers for 25 to 30 minutes, or until they are soft.

- Remove the foil and bake for an additional 5-10 minutes to melt the cheese.

- Serve hot.

2. Lentil and Vegetable Stir-Fry

Ingredients:

- 1 cup green or brown lentils, cooked

- 2 cups mixed vegetables (broccoli, bell peppers, carrots), chopped

- 1 onion, thinly sliced

- 2 cloves garlic, minced

- 2 tablespoons soy sauce (low-sodium)

- 1 tablespoon sesame oil

- 1 teaspoon ginger, minced

- 1 teaspoon sesame seeds

- Salt and pepper to taste

Instructions:

- In a sizable pan or wok, heat the sesame oil over medium heat.

- Add sliced onion, minced garlic, and minced ginger. Sauté until fragrant.

- Add chopped mixed vegetables and cook until slightly tender.

- Stir in cooked lentils and soy sauce. Cook for a few more minutes.

- Season with salt and pepper.
- Garnish with sesame seeds before serving.

3. *Mushroom and Spinach Risotto*

Ingredients:

- 1 cup Arborio rice
- 4 cups vegetable broth
- 1 cup mushrooms, sliced
- 2 cups baby spinach
- 1 onion, chopped
- 2 cloves garlic, minced
- ½ cup dry white wine (optional)
- ¼ cup nutritional yeast
- 2 tablespoons olive oil
- Salt and pepper to taste

Instructions:

- In a saucepan, heat vegetable broth and keep it warm.

- In a large pan, sauté chopped onion and minced garlic in olive oil until translucent.

- Arborio rice should be added and cooked for a few minutes until just lightly toasted.

- If using wine, pour it into the pan and cook until absorbed.

- Gradually add warm vegetable broth, ½ cup at a time, stirring frequently until absorbed before adding more.

- Stir in sliced mushrooms and continue adding broth until the rice is creamy and cooked.

- Add baby spinach and nutritional yeast. Cook until the spinach wilts.

- Season with salt and pepper.

- Serve hot.

4 Chickpea and Vegetable Curry

Ingredients:

- 2 cups cooked chickpeas

- 2 cups mixed vegetables (zucchini, bell peppers, peas), chopped

- 1 onion, chopped

- 2 cloves garlic, minced

- 1 can (14 oz) diced tomatoes

- 1 can (14 oz) coconut milk

- 2 tablespoons curry powder

- 1 teaspoon turmeric

- 1 teaspoon ground cumin

- 1 teaspoon paprika

- 1 tablespoon olive oil

- Fresh cilantro for garnish

- Salt and pepper to taste

Instructions:

- In a large pan, sauté chopped onion and minced garlic in olive oil until translucent.

- Add curry powder, turmeric, ground cumin, and paprika. Stir for a minute.

- Add chopped mixed vegetables and cook until slightly tender.

- Pour in diced tomatoes (with juices) and coconut milk.

- Stir in cooked chickpeas and let the curry simmer for 10-15 minutes.

- Season with salt and pepper.

- Garnish with fresh cilantro before serving.

5. *Mediterranean Stuffed Portobello Mushrooms*

Ingredients:

- 4 large portobello mushrooms, stems removed

- 1 cup cooked quinoa

- 1 cup diced tomatoes

- ½ cup chopped Kalamata olives

- ½ cup crumbled feta cheese (vegan if preferred)

- ¼ cup chopped fresh parsley

- 2 tablespoons balsamic vinegar

- 2 tablespoons olive oil

- Salt and pepper to taste

Instructions:

- Preheat the oven to 375°F (190°C).

- In a bowl, combine cooked quinoa, diced tomatoes, chopped Kalamata olives, crumbled feta cheese, chopped fresh parsley, balsamic vinegar, olive oil, salt, and pepper.

- The portobello mushrooms should be put on a baking sheet.

- Fill each mushroom cap with the quinoa mixture.

- Bake the mushrooms for 20 to 25 minutes, or until they are soft.

- Serve hot.

6. Roasted Vegetable and Hummus Wrap

Ingredients:

- 2 whole wheat tortillas

- 1 cup hummus

- 2 cups mixed roasted vegetables (bell peppers, zucchini, eggplant), sliced

- 1 cup baby spinach

- ¼ cup red onion, thinly sliced

- 2 tablespoons balsamic glaze

- Salt and pepper to taste

Instructions:

- Spread hummus evenly on each whole wheat tortilla.

- Arrange mixed roasted vegetables, baby spinach, and red onion slices on top.

- Drizzle with balsamic glaze.

- Season with salt and pepper.

- Roll up the tortillas, securing the filling.

- Serve as wraps.

7. *Lentil and Vegetable Casserole*

- **Ingredients:**

- 1 cup green or brown lentils, cooked

- 2 cups mixed vegetables (carrots, peas, corn), cooked

- 1 onion, chopped

- 2 cloves garlic, minced

- 1 can (14 oz) diced tomatoes

- 1 teaspoon dried oregano

- 1 teaspoon dried basil

- ½ teaspoon red pepper flakes (optional)

- 1 cup shredded vegan cheese

- Salt and pepper to taste

Instructions:

- Preheat the oven to 375°F (190°C).

- In a pan, sauté chopped onion and minced garlic until translucent.

- Add diced tomatoes, dried oregano, dried basil, and red pepper flakes. Simmer for a few minutes.

- Layer cooked lentils and mixed vegetables in a baking dish.

- Pour the tomato mixture over the lentil and vegetable layers.

- Sprinkle shredded vegan cheese on top.

- Bake for 20 to 25 minutes, or until the cheese is bubbling and melted.

- Serve hot.

8. Spinach and Tofu Stir-Fry

Ingredients:

- 1 block (14 oz) firm tofu, cubed

- 4 cups fresh baby spinach

- 1 red bell pepper, sliced

- 1 carrot, julienned

- 2 cloves garlic, minced

- 2 tablespoons low-sodium soy sauce

- 1 tablespoon sesame oil

- 1 teaspoon ginger, minced

- 1 teaspoon sesame seeds

- Salt and pepper to taste

Instructions:

- In a large pan, heat sesame oil over medium heat.

- Add cubed tofu and cook until lightly golden on all sides. Set aside.

- In the same pan, sauté sliced red bell pepper, julienned carrot, minced garlic, and minced ginger until vegetables are slightly tender.

- Add cooked tofu and fresh baby spinach. Stir-fry until spinach is wilted.

- Drizzle low-sodium soy sauce over the stir-fry.

- Season with salt, pepper, and sesame seeds.

- Serve hot.

9. Butternut Squash and Chickpea Stew

Ingredients:

- 3 cups butternut squash, cubed

- 1 can (14 oz) drained and rinsed chickpeas

- 1 onion, chopped

- 2 cloves garlic, minced

- 1 can (14 oz) diced tomatoes

- 4 cups vegetable broth

- 1 teaspoon ground cumin

- 1 teaspoon ground coriander

- ½ teaspoon ground cinnamon

- ¼ teaspoon red pepper flakes (optional)

- 2 tablespoons olive oil

- Fresh cilantro for garnish

- Salt and pepper to taste

Instructions:

- In a pot, sauté chopped onion and minced garlic in olive oil until translucent.

- Add cubed butternut squash and sauté for a few minutes.

- Stir in ground cumin, ground coriander, ground cinnamon, and red pepper flakes.

- Pour in diced tomatoes (with juices) and vegetable broth. Simmer until butternut squash is tender.

- Add drained chickpeas and simmer for another 10-15 minutes.

- Season with salt and pepper.

- Garnish with fresh cilantro before serving.

10. Eggplant Parmesan

Ingredients:

- 2 large eggplants, sliced into rounds

- 2 cups marinara sauce (store-bought or homemade)

- 2 cups shredded vegan mozzarella cheese

- 1 cup breadcrumbs (gluten-free if preferred)

- ½ cup nutritional yeast

- ¼ cup fresh basil leaves, chopped

- 2 tablespoons olive oil

- Salt and pepper to taste

Instructions:

- Preheat the oven to 375°F (190°C).

- Dip eggplant slices in olive oil, then coat with breadcrumbs mixed with nutritional yeast.

- Place the coated eggplant slices on a baking sheet and bake for about 20 minutes, until golden and crispy.

- Spread a layer of marinara sauce in a baking dish.

- Layer baked eggplant slices, followed by shredded vegan mozzarella cheese and chopped basil.

- Repeat the layers until all ingredients are used, finishing with a layer of cheese and basil on top.

- Until the cheese is melted and bubbling, bake for 20 to 25 minutes.

- Serve hot.

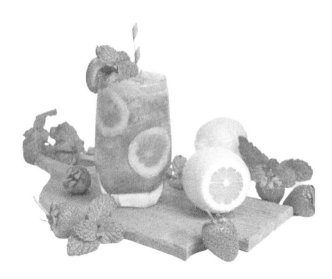

Chapter Six

Satisfying Cravings: Vegetarian Galveston Snacks and Appetizer Creations

1. Avocado Hummus Dip

Ingredients:

- 1 ripe avocado
- 1 cup cooked chickpeas
- 2 tablespoons lemon juice
- 1 clove garlic
- 2 tablespoons olive oil
- Salt and pepper to taste

Instructions:

- Blend avocado, chickpeas, lemon juice, garlic, and olive oil until smooth.

- Season with salt and pepper. Serve with veggie sticks.

2. *Cucumber Bites with Greek Yogurt*

Ingredients:

- Cucumber slices

- 1/2 cup Greek yogurt

- 1 teaspoon dill

- Cherry tomatoes

- Black olives

Instructions:

- Mix Greek yogurt with dill. Top cucumber slices with yogurt mixture.

- Garnish with cherry tomatoes and black olives.

3. *Stuffed Bell Pepper Poppers*

Ingredients:

- Mini bell peppers

- 1/2 cup cream cheese

- 1/4 cup chopped spinach

- 1/4 cup shredded cheddar cheese

Instructions:

- Mix cream cheese and chopped spinach.

- Stuff mini bell peppers with the mixture and sprinkle with cheddar cheese.

4. Roasted Chickpeas

Ingredients:

- 1 cup cooked chickpeas

- 1 tablespoon olive oil

- 1 teaspoon paprika

- 1/2 teaspoon cumin

- 1/2 teaspoon garlic powder

Instructions:

- Toss chickpeas with olive oil and spices.

- Roast in the oven at 400°F (200°C) for 20-25 minutes, until crispy.

5. *Zucchini Fritters*

Ingredients:

- 2 cups grated zucchini

- 1/4 cup flour (or almond flour for gluten-free)

- 1 egg (or a flax egg if you're vegan)

- 1/4 cup finely chopped onion

- 2 cloves garlic, minced

- 2 tablespoons chopped fresh herbs (such as parsley and dill)

Instructions:

- Mix grated zucchini with flour, egg, onion, garlic, and herbs.

- Form into patties and cook in a pan with a drizzle of olive oil until golden on both sides.

6. Guacamole-Stuffed Cherry Tomatoes

Ingredients:

- Cherry tomatoes

- 2 ripe avocados

- 2 tablespoons finely diced red onion

- 1 tablespoon lime juice

- 2 tablespoons chopped cilantro

- Salt and pepper to taste

Instructions:

- Cut tops off cherry tomatoes and scoop out the insides.

- Mash avocados and mix with red onion, lime juice, cilantro, salt, and pepper.

- Fill cherry tomatoes with guacamole.

7. Spinach and Artichoke Dip

Ingredients:

- 1 cup chopped spinach (cooked and drained)

- 1/2 cup canned artichoke hearts, chopped

- 1/2 cup Greek yogurt

- 1/4 cup grated Parmesan cheese

- 1 clove garlic, minced

- Salt and pepper to taste

Instructions:

- Mix chopped spinach, artichoke hearts, Greek yogurt, Parmesan cheese, and garlic.

- Season with salt and pepper. Serve with whole-grain crackers.

8. Cucumber and Hummus Roll-Ups

Ingredients:

- Cucumber slices

- Hummus

- Sliced bell peppers

- Baby spinach leaves

Instructions:

- Spread hummus on cucumber slices.

- Top with bell pepper slices and baby spinach. Roll up and secure with toothpicks.

9. Greek Salad Skewers

Ingredients:

- Cherry tomatoes

- Cucumber chunks

- Kalamata olives

- Feta cheese

- Drizzle of olive oil and sprinkle of oregano

Instructions:

- Thread cherry tomatoes, cucumbers, olives, and feta onto skewers.

- Sprinkle some oregano and drizzle with olive oil.

10. Fruit Kabobs with Yogurt Dip

Ingredients:

- Assorted fruits (berries, melon, grapes)

- 1 cup Greek yogurt

- 2 tablespoons honey

- 1 teaspoon vanilla extract

Instructions:

- Thread fruits onto skewers.

- Mix Greek yogurt with honey and vanilla extract for dip.

Chapter Seven

Staying Hydrated and Nourished with Flavorful Beverages

1. Green Goddess Smoothie

Ingredients:

- 1 cup spinach leaves

- 1/2 banana

- 1/2 cup cucumber, chopped

- 1/2 cup unsweetened almond milk

- 1/4 avocado

- 1 tablespoon chia seeds

- Ice cubes

Instructions:

- Blend every ingredient until it is creamy and smooth.

- Add more almond milk if needed for desired consistency.

2. *Tropical Turmeric Cooler*

Ingredients:

- 1 cup pineapple chunks

- 1/2 banana

- 1/2 teaspoon turmeric powder

- 1/2 teaspoon grated ginger

- 1 cup coconut water

- Ice cubes

Instructions:

- Blend pineapple, banana, turmeric, ginger, and coconut water until well combined.

- Add ice cubes. Blend again until chilled and smooth.

3. Cucumber Mint Refresher

Ingredients:

- 1 cucumber, peeled and chopped
- Handful of fresh mint leaves
- Juice of 1 lime
- 1 cup water
- Ice cubes

Instructions:

- Blend cucumber, mint leaves, lime juice, and water until smooth.
- Add ice cubes and blend again until chilled.

4. Berry Blast Smoothie

Ingredients:

- 1/2 cup mixed berries (strawberries, blueberries, raspberries)
- 1/2 banana

- 1/2 cup unsweetened almond milk

- 1 tablespoon chia seeds

- Ice cubes

Instructions:

- Blend mixed berries, banana, almond milk, and chia seeds until well blended.

- Add ice cubes and blend until smooth.

5. *Golden Milk Latte*

Ingredients:

- 1 cup unsweetened almond milk

- 1/2 teaspoon turmeric powder

- 1/4 teaspoon cinnamon

- Pinch of black pepper

- 1 teaspoon maple syrup (optional)

Instructions:

- In a saucepan over medium heat, heat the almond milk.

- Add turmeric, cinnamon, black pepper, and maple syrup (if using).

- Whisk until well combined and heated through. Do not boil.

6. Citrus Splash Infused Water

Ingredients:

- Slices of orange, lemon, and lime

- Fresh mint leaves

- 1 liter water

Instructions:

- In a pitcher, combine slices of citrus fruits and fresh mint leaves.

- Fill the pitcher with water and refrigerate for a few hours before serving.

7. Watermelon Cooler

Ingredients:

- 2 cups cubed watermelon
- 1/2 lime, juiced
- 1/4 cup fresh basil leaves
- 1 cup coconut water
- Ice cubes

Instructions:

- Blend watermelon, lime juice, basil leaves, and coconut water until smooth.
- Add ice cubes and blend until chilled.

8. *Herbal Iced Tea*

Ingredients:

- 2 herbal tea bags (such as chamomile, peppermint, or ginger)
- 1 liter water
- Slices of lemon or orange (optional)
- Honey or stevia to taste (optional)

Instructions:

- Boil water and steep the herbal tea bags for about 5 minutes.

- Let the tea cool, then refrigerate until cold.

- Serve over ice with slices of lemon or orange and sweeten with honey or stevia if desired.

9. Creamy Cashew Milkshake

Ingredients:

- 1/4 cup raw cashews, soaked and drained

- 1 cup unsweetened almond milk

- 1/2 banana

- 1 tablespoon cacao powder or cocoa powder

- 1/2 teaspoon vanilla extract

- Ice cubes

Instructions:

- Blend soaked cashews, almond milk, banana, cacao powder, and vanilla extract until creamy.

- Add ice cubes and blend until chilled and frothy.

10. Berry Hibiscus Iced Tea

Ingredients:

- 2 hibiscus tea bags

- 1/2 cup mixed berries (strawberries, blueberries, raspberries)

- 1 liter water

- Honey or stevia to taste (optional)

Instructions:

- Boil water and steep the hibiscus tea bags for about 5 minutes.

- Let the tea cool, then refrigerate until cold.

- In a glass, muddle the mixed berries, then pour in the hibiscus tea.

- Sweeten with honey or stevia if desired.

Chapter Eight

Bowlfuls of Goodness: Satisfying Vegetarian Galveston Diet Soups

1. Creamy Broccoli Soup

Ingredients:

- 2 cups broccoli florets

- 1 onion, chopped

- 2 garlic cloves, minced

- 2 cups vegetable broth

- 1 cup almond milk

- Salt and pepper to taste

Instructions:

- In a pot, sauté the chopped onion and minced garlic until fragrant.

- Add the broccoli florets and cook for a few minutes.

- Add the veggie broth, and then simmer.

- Once the broccoli is tender, use an immersion blender to puree the soup until smooth.

- Stir in almond milk and season with salt and pepper.

- Simmer for a few more minutes and adjust seasoning as needed. Serve warm.

2. Lentil and Spinach Soup

Ingredients:

- 1 cup red lentils, rinsed

- 1 onion, chopped

- 2 carrots, diced

- 2 cups fresh spinach

- 6 cups vegetable broth

- 1 tsp cumin

- Salt and pepper to taste

Instructions:

- In a large pot, sauté the chopped onion until translucent.

- Add the diced carrots and cook for a few minutes.

- Add the red lentils, cumin, and vegetable broth. Bring to a boil.

- Reduce heat and let simmer until lentils are cooked.

- Stir in fresh spinach and let it wilt.

- Season with salt and pepper. Serve hot.

3. Roasted Red Pepper Soup

Ingredients:

- 3 red bell peppers, roasted and peeled

- 1 onion, chopped

- 2 garlic cloves, minced

- 4 cups vegetable broth

- 1 can (14 oz) diced tomatoes

- 1 tsp paprika

- Salt and pepper to taste

Instructions:

- The minced garlic and diced onion should be sautéed in a pot until soft.

- Add the roasted red peppers, diced tomatoes, and vegetable broth.

- Simmer for about 15 minutes.

- Until the soup is creamy, purée it using an immersion blender.

- Add paprika, salt, and pepper. Simmer for a few more minutes. Serve warm.

4. Butternut Squash Soup

Ingredients:

- 1 butternut squash, peeled and cubed

- 1 onion, chopped

- 2 carrots, diced

- 4 cups vegetable broth

- 1 tsp cinnamon

- 1/2 tsp nutmeg

- Salt and pepper to taste

Instructions:

- In a large pot, sauté the chopped onion until translucent.

- Add the diced carrots and cubed butternut squash. Cook for a few minutes.

- Add the veggie broth, then bring to a simmer.

- Let the vegetables cook until tender.

- Until the soup is smooth, blend it using an immersion blender.

- Add cinnamon, nutmeg, salt, and pepper. Simmer for a few more minutes. Serve hot.

5. *Coconut Curry Chickpea Soup*

Ingredients:

- A can (15 oz) chickpeas (drained and rinsed)

- 1 onion, chopped

- 2 garlic cloves, minced

- 1 can (14 oz) coconut milk

- 2 cups vegetable broth

- 2 tsp curry powder

- 1 tsp turmeric

- Salt and pepper to taste

Instructions:

- In a pot, sauté the chopped onion and minced garlic until fragrant.

- Add the chickpeas, curry powder, and turmeric. Cook for a few minutes.

- Pour in the coconut milk and vegetable broth. Bring to a simmer.

- Let the flavors meld together for about 10 minutes.

- Season with salt and pepper. Serve warm.

6. Mushroom and Barley Soup

Ingredients:

- 2 cups mushrooms, sliced

- 1 onion, chopped

- 2 carrots, diced

- 1 cup barley, rinsed

- 6 cups vegetable broth

- 2 tsp thyme

- Salt and pepper to taste

Instructions:

- In a large pot, sauté the chopped onion until translucent.

- Add the sliced mushrooms and diced carrots. Cook until softened.

- Stir in the rinsed barley and vegetable broth. Bring to a boil.

- Reduce the heat and allow the barley to simmer until it is tender.

- Add thyme, salt, and pepper. Simmer for a few more minutes. Serve hot.

7. Spinach and Quinoa Soup

Ingredients:

- 1 cup quinoa, rinsed

- 2 cups fresh spinach

- 1 onion, chopped

- 2 garlic cloves, minced

- 6 cups vegetable broth

- 1 tsp dried oregano

- Salt and pepper to taste

Instructions:

- In a pot, sauté the chopped onion and minced garlic until fragrant.

- Add the rinsed quinoa and dried oregano. Cook for a few minutes.

- The vegetable broth should be poured in and brought to a boil.

- Reduce the heat and let the quinoa cook until tender.

- Stir in fresh spinach and let it wilt.

- Season with salt and pepper. Serve warm.

8. Zucchini and Potato Soup

Ingredients:

- 2 zucchinis, diced

- 2 potatoes, peeled and diced

- 1 onion, chopped

- 4 cups vegetable broth

- 1 tsp thyme

- Salt and pepper to taste

Instructions:

- In a large pot, sauté the chopped onion until translucent.

- Add the diced zucchinis and potatoes. Cook for a few minutes.

- Pour in the vegetable broth, then bring to a simmer.

- Let the vegetables cook until tender.

- Add thyme, salt, and pepper. Simmer for a few more minutes. Serve hot.

9. Tuscan White Bean Soup

Ingredients:

- 1 can (15 oz) drained and rinsed white beans

- 1 onion, chopped

- 2 carrots, diced

- 2 celery stalks, diced

- 4 cups vegetable broth

- 1 can (14 oz) diced tomatoes

- 1 tsp rosemary

- Salt and pepper to taste

Instructions:

- In a pot, sauté the chopped onion until translucent.

- Add the diced carrots and celery. Cook for a few minutes.

- Stir in the white beans, diced tomatoes, and vegetable broth.

- Bring to a simmer and let the flavors meld for about 15 minutes.

- Add rosemary, salt, and pepper. Simmer for a few more minutes. Serve warm.

10. Spicy Black Bean Soup

Ingredients:

- 2 cans (15 oz each) black beans, drained and rinsed

- 1 onion, chopped

- 2 bell peppers, diced

- 2 garlic cloves, minced

- 4 cups vegetable broth

- 1 tsp cumin

- 1/2 tsp chili powder

- Salt and pepper to taste

Instructions:

- The minced garlic and diced onion should be cooked until aromatic in a big pot.

- The diced bell peppers should be added and cooked until tender.

- Stir in the black beans, cumin, and chili powder. Cook for a few minutes.

- Add the veggie broth, and then simmer.

- For about 15 minutes, let the flavors meld together.

- Season with salt and pepper. Serve hot.

Chapter Nine

28-Day Guide: Your Vegetarian Galveston Diet Meal Plan

Week 1: Energizing Beginnings

Day 1:

- Breakfast: Green smoothie (banana, almond milk, spinach, chia seeds)

- Lunch: Quinoa salad with mixed vegetables and lemon-tahini dressing

- Dinner: A side of mixed greens with lentil soup

- Snack: Greek yogurt with berries

Day 2:

- Breakfast: Oatmeal topped with sliced almonds and berries

- Lunch: Chickpea salad with cucumber, tomato, red onion, and feta cheese

- Dinner: Zucchini noodles with marinara sauce and a side salad

- Snack: Hummus and veggie sticks

Day 3:

- Breakfast: Greek yogurt with chopped nuts and honey

- Lunch: Hummus and avocado wrap with whole wheat tortilla

- Dinner: Stuffed bell peppers with rice, black beans, and veggies

- Snack: Apple slices with almond butter

Day 4:

- Breakfast: Whole grain toast and spinach with scrambled tofu

- Lunch: Black bean bowl and quinoa with salsa and avocado

- Dinner: Eggplant Parmesan with a side of roasted Brussels sprouts

- Snack: Rice cakes with peanut butter

Day 5:

- Breakfast: Almond milk, granola, and mixed berries in a smoothie bowl

- Lunch: Mediterranean salad with olives, cucumber, tomato, and feta cheese

- Dinner: Tofu and brown rice with vegetable stir-fry

- Snack: Trail mix with dried fruit and nuts

Day 6:

- Breakfast: Chia seed pudding with almond milk and fresh fruit

- Lunch: Spinach and feta stuffed portobello mushrooms

- Dinner: Lentil curry with quinoa

- Snack: Carrot and celery sticks with hummus

Day 7:

- Breakfast: Whole grain pancakes with maple syrup

- Lunch: Caprese salad with basil, tomato, and mozzarella

- Dinner: Sweet potato and black bean enchiladas

- Snack: Cottage cheese with pineapple

Week 2: Nourishing Discoveries

Day 8:

- Breakfast: Nut butter and banana sandwich on whole grain bread

- Lunch: Roasted vegetable and hummus wrap

- Dinner: Acorn squash stuffed with cranberries and wild rice

- Snack: Rice crackers with cheese

Day 9:

- Breakfast: Berry and nut granola parfait with yogurt

- Lunch: Greek quinoa salad with olives, cucumber, tomato, and feta cheese

- Dinner: Veggie burger with a side salad

- Snack: Mixed nuts

Day 10:

- Breakfast: Fruit salad with mixed fruits and honey

- Lunch: Mediterranean hummus and vegetable wrap

- Dinner: Cauliflower rice stir-fry with mixed vegetables and tofu

- Snack: Rice cakes with almond butter

Day 11:

- Breakfast: Smoothie with banana, kale and almond milk

- Lunch: Spinach and strawberry salad with goat cheese and balsamic dressing

- Dinner: Ratatouille with a side of quinoa

- Snack: Greek yogurt with walnuts

Day 12:

- Breakfast: Veggie omelette with tomatoes, bell peppers, and onions

- Lunch: Black bean and corn salad with lime vinaigrette

- Dinner: Lentil and vegetable stew

- Snack: Fruit and cheese platter

Day 13:

- Breakfast: Whole grain waffles with fresh berries

- Lunch: Caprese quinoa salad with mozzarella, tomato, and basil

- Dinner: Vegetable and chickpea coconut curry with brown rice

- Snack: Veggie chips with salsa

Day 14:

- Breakfast: Nut butter and banana smoothie

- Lunch: Chickpea and avocado salad

- Dinner: Mushroom and spinach pasta with garlic bread

- Snack: Edamame beans

Week 3: Balanced Delights

Day 15:

- Breakfast: Overnight oats with almond milk, chia seeds, and dried fruit

- Lunch: Roasted vegetable and quinoa bowl with tahini dressing

- Dinner: Zucchini noodles with pesto and cherry tomatoes

- Snack: Rice cakes with hummus

Day 16:

- Breakfast: Almonds and sliced peaches with cottage cheese

- Lunch: Hummus and roasted vegetable wrap

- Dinner: Lentil and sweet potato stew

- Snack: Apple slices with nut butter

Day 17:

- Breakfast: Spinach and whole grain toast with scrambled tofu

- Lunch: Mediterranean couscous salad with olives, cucumber, and feta cheese

- Dinner: Stuffed mushrooms with quinoa and herbs

- Snack: Trail mix with dried fruit

Day 18:

- Breakfast: Greek yogurt with honey and mixed nuts

- Lunch: Spinach and white bean salad with lemon-tahini dressing

- Dinner: Vegetable and tofu stir-fry with brown rice

- Snack: Rice crackers with cheese

Day 19:

- Breakfast: Chia seed pudding with almond milk and fresh fruit

- Lunch: Hummus and avocado wrap with whole wheat tortilla

- Dinner: Eggplant and spinach lasagna

- Snack: Carrot and celery sticks with hummus

Day 20:

- Breakfast: Smoothie bowl with almond milk, granola, and mixed berries

- Lunch: Salsa and avocado with black bean bow and quinoa

- Dinner: Vegetable and lentil curry with rice

- Snack: Mixed nuts

Day 21:

- Breakfast: Blueberry almond smoothie with spinach and chia seeds

- Lunch: Chickpea and quinoa salad with mixed vegetables and lemon dressing

- Dinner: Wild rice and cranberries with stuffed acorn squash

- Snack: Handful of mixed nuts

Week 4: Vibrant Culmination

Day 22:

- Breakfast: Scrambled tofu with spinach and tomatoes

- Lunch: Chickpea and brown rice with vegetable stir-fry

- Dinner: Vegetable stew with whole-grain bread and lentils

- Snack: Greek yogurt with mixed berries

Day 23:

- Breakfast: Smoothie with mixed berries, spinach, banana, and almond milk

- Lunch: Roasted vegetables and lemon-tahini dressing with quinoa salad

- Dinner: Stuffed bell peppers with black beans, quinoa, and salsa

- Snack: Apple slices with almond butter

Day 24:

- Breakfast: Almond milk, chia seeds, and sliced almonds with overnight oats.

- Lunch: Spinach and avocado salad with chickpeas and balsamic vinaigrette

- Dinner: Vegetable curry with tofu and brown rice

- Snack: Carrot and cucumber sticks with hummus

Day 25:

- Breakfast: Greek yogurt parfait with granola and mixed fruit

- Lunch: Mediterranean quinoa bowl with olives, cucumber, tomato, and feta cheese

- Dinner: Portobello mushroom burgers with sweet potato fries

- Snack: Trail mix with nuts and dried fruits

Day 26:

- Breakfast: Whole-grain toast with smashed avocado and cherry tomatoes

- Lunch: Lentil and vegetable wrap with a side salad

- Dinner: Zucchini noodles with pesto and cherry tomatoes

- Snack: Rice cakes with almond butter and banana slices

Day 27:

- Breakfast: Oatmeal with mixed nuts, dried fruits, and a drizzle of honey

- Lunch: Hummus and vegetable wrap with a side of mixed greens

- Dinner: Roasted vegetable and quinoa stuffed bell peppers

- Snack: Rice crackers with guacamole

Day 28:

- Breakfast: Chia seed pudding with coconut flakes and fresh berries

- Lunch: Mozzarella, tomatoes, basil, and balsamic glaze in a caprese salad

- Dinner: Spinach and mushroom frittata with a side of mixed greens

- Snack: Sliced pear with cottage chees

Please adjust portion sizes and ingredients according to your preferences and dietary needs. Before making any dietary changes, always speak with a healthcare provider, especially if you have underlying medical issues.

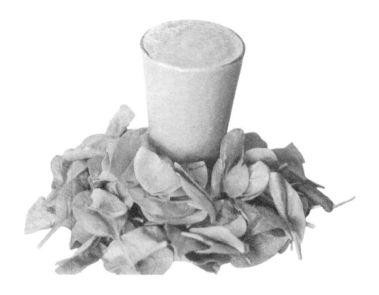

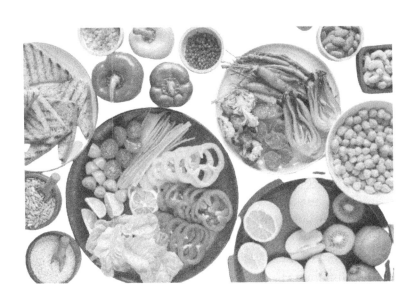

Chapter 10

Glowing Wellness: Lifestyle Strategies for Your Vegetarian Galveston Diet Success

Adopting a successful vegetarian Galveston lifestyle is a comprehensive endeavor that encompasses various aspects of well-being. These tips and strategies provide a detailed look into creating a balanced and fulfilling lifestyle tailored to your dietary preferences and health goals.

Mindful Meal Planning: Craft a well-thought-out meal plan that includes a wide range of plant-based foods. This approach ensures you receive a spectrum of nutrients necessary for optimal health. Prioritize leafy greens, colorful vegetables, whole grains, and a variety of legumes to create nutrient-rich and satisfying meals.

Hydration is Key: Water plays a vital role in maintaining bodily functions, including digestion. Aim to drink an adequate amount of water throughout the day to stay hydrated and support the digestive process.

Choose Nutrient-Rich Foods: Select foods that provide essential vitamins, minerals, and antioxidants. These elements contribute to overall well-being and promote a strong immune system.

Balanced Macro-nutrients: Balance your meals by incorporating complex carbohydrates, healthy fats, and quality proteins. This combination stabilizes blood sugar levels, provides sustained energy, and supports optimal digestion.

Portion Control: Portion control is important to avoid overeating, which can strain the digestive system.Utilize visual cues like your hand size to gauge appropriate portion sizes.

Include High-Fiber Foods: Fiber is instrumental in maintaining digestive health. Fiber-rich foods such as whole grains, legumes, vegetables, and fruits facilitate regular bowel movements and foster a diverse gut microbiome.

Mindful Eating: Eat with intention and awareness. Savor each bite, chew thoroughly, and pay attention to hunger and fullness cues. Mindful eating enhances digestion by allowing your body to process food effectively.

Stay Active: Regular physical activity supports a healthy digestive system. Engage in exercises you enjoy, whether it's brisk walking, yoga, or swimming, to enhance overall well-being.

Manage Stress: Stress can disrupt digestion. Incorporate stress-relief practices like deep breathing, meditation, and gentle stretching into your routine to foster a calm and balanced state.

Probiotics and Prebiotics: Optimize gut health by including probiotic-rich foods (such as fermented yogurts, kefir, and kimchi) and prebiotic foods (like garlic, onions, and asparagus) in your diet. Digestion is more effective when the gut is in balance.

Limit Processed Foods: Reduce processed and sugary foods in your diet. These items can irritate the gut lining and lead to digestive discomfort.

Cook at Home: Preparing meals at home offers control over ingredients and cooking methods. Experiment with new recipes and ingredients to keep your meals exciting and nourishing.

Stay Consistent: Consistency is key to establishing lasting habits. Stick to your vegetarian Galveston lifestyle plan, even on busy days, to maintain the positive impact on your digestive health.

Stay Hydrated: Prioritize water consumption and incorporate herbal teas into your routine. Adequate hydration supports digestion and overall well-being.

Sleep Well: Prioritize quality sleep to allow your body to rejuvenate and restore its natural functions, including digestion.

Social Support: Join vegetarian groups, forums, or local meetups to connect with like-minded individuals. Sharing experiences, recipes, and challenges can provide encouragement and inspiration.

Educate Yourself: Stay informed about vegetarian nutrition, culinary techniques, and the benefits of a Galveston-inspired lifestyle. Continuous learning empowers you to make informed choices.

Celebrate Progress: Acknowledge your achievements and milestones, no matter how small. Celebrating your progress boosts motivation and reinforces positive habits.

Consult a Professional: If you have unique health concerns or dietary needs, consider seeking guidance from a registered dietitian or healthcare professional. Their expertise can provide personalized recommendations.

Stay Positive: Embrace a positive attitude towards your journey. Believe in your ability to create a flourishing vegetarian Galveston lifestyle that nurtures both your body and mind.

By integrating these strategies into your daily life, you're nurturing a lifestyle that supports digestive wellness, enhances overall health, and enriches your quality of life.

Conclusion

Embrace the Vegetarian Galveston Way for Lifelong Wellness

As you close the pages of this cookbook, you're not just ending a culinary adventure, but you're embarking on a lifelong journey of health and wellness through the vegetarian Galveston diet. With each recipe you've explored and every tip you've absorbed, you've gained the tools to create a balanced and nourishing lifestyle that will serve you well for years to come.

The recipes within these pages are more than just a collection of dishes; they are a testament to your commitment to embracing wholesome, plant-based nutrition. By incorporating these flavors into your meals, you've not only catered to your taste buds but also paved the way for a healthier and more vibrant you.

The lifestyle tips you've encountered provide a roadmap for sustainable well-being. From mindful eating practices to self-care routines, you've discovered how small changes can make a big impact on your overall health. By choosing the vegetarian Galveston approach, you've demonstrated that wellness is a choice you actively make every day.

As you continue your journey, remember that this cookbook is a starting point, not a destination. Use these recipes and tips as a foundation to create your own culinary masterpieces and cultivate a lifestyle that aligns with your health goals.

With gratitude for joining us on this transformative path, we encourage you to carry the spirit of the vegetarian Galveston diet into your everyday life. Embrace the nourishing power of plant-based foods, and may your journey be filled with vibrant health, satisfaction, and the joy of living life to the fullest.

Weekly Meal Planner

Monday

Tuesday

Wednesday

Thursday

Friday

Saturday

Sunday

Notes

Weekly Meal Planner

Monday

Tuesday

Wednesday

Thursday

Friday

Saturday

Sunday

Notes

Weekly Meal Planner

Monday

Tuesday

Wednesday

Thursday

Friday

Saturday

Sunday

Notes

Weekly Meal Planner

Monday

Tuesday

Wednesday

Thursday

Friday

Saturday

Sunday

Notes

Weekly Meal Planner

Monday

Tuesday

Wednesday

Thursday

Friday

Saturday

Sunday

Notes

Weekly Meal Planner

Monday

Tuesday

Wednesday

Thursday

Friday

Saturday

Sunday

Notes

Weekly Meal Planner

Monday

Tuesday

Wednesday

Thursday

Friday

Saturday

Sunday

Notes

Weekly Meal Planner

Monday

Tuesday

Wednesday

Thursday

Friday

Saturday

Sunday

Notes

Weekly Meal Planner

Monday

Tuesday

Wednesday

Thursday

Friday

Saturday

Sunday

Notes

Weekly Meal Planner

Monday

Tuesday

Wednesday

Thursday

Friday

Saturday

Sunday

Notes

Made in the USA
Las Vegas, NV
23 June 2024

91386331R00069